D1561988

Trigger Finger Cure

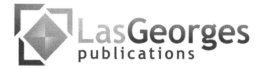

Trigger Finger Cure

Joshua L. Sho

Foreword by Professor Rana K. Williamson

Edited By Brenda McPhersons

Cover Design by Dr. Jay Polma

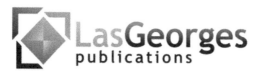

UNITED KINGDOM

LasGEORGES Publications 49, Telford Drive,
Slough SL1 9LB United Kingdom

This paperback was first published in Great Britain
in 2013 by LasGEORGES Publications
www.LasGEORGESPublications.com
Copyright © LasGEORGES Publications 2013

LasGEORGES Publications has asserted the right
under the Copyright, Designs and Patent Act 1988
to be the owner of this work.

Cover Designed by Dr. Jay Polma

All Products, publications, software and services
Mentioned and recommended in this publication are protected by trademarks.
In such instance, all Trademark & Copyright belong to the respective owners.

A CIP catalogue record of this book is available from the British Library.

ISBN 978-0-9575791-2-5
Publisher Number 978-0-9575791

**Printed and bound in Great Britain
by Lightning Source UK Ltd, Milton Keynes. UK**

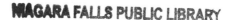

Contents

Acknowledgements

I am Grateful to the many people who encouraged me, believed me, supported and helped to make this publication a reality. My Deepest thanks to my very good friend Professor Rana K. Williamson for writing the foreword to this comprehensive guide, to Brenda McPhersons for editing the book and Dr. Jay Polma for designing the cover page.

I also like to acknowledge the following people for their invaluable assistance in helping me to research and write one of the most comprehensive and up-to-date book on this topic. I thank them for their insight, patience, and professional input. Just to mention a few; Neil Armstrong, Graeme Oxford, Nicky Nelson, Jacob Fletcher, Harvey Carol, Richard Flack and many others. Thank you all.

Foreword by Dr. Rana K. Williamson

What do you do? Your friend says, "I'm going to write a book about trigger finger." In my case, my eyes glazed over a bit, and I murmured something along the lines of, "That's great, Joshua!" At the same time, I suspect I was praying I didn't get asked to read the book.

My prayers weren't answered. I did get asked to read the book. To say that I was pleasantly surprised is an understatement. I found myself not only interested, but intrigued by the fact that so many diverse conditions can manifest in locked joints.

It's clear that "classic" trigger finger is a predictable mechanical malfunction, but there are so many other reasons the problem can surface, some even tied to diet. That's an area of particular interest to me as a vegan, and what I read here makes absolute sense. The modern diet, especially in America is a disaster. If our bodies can't get our attention one way, they'll get it another.

This is an easily accessible overview of what can be a medically dense subject. Even the proper name for trigger finger, "stenosing tenosynovitis" is a tongue twister.

Without getting into intricate fine points of anatomy, Joshua explains classic trigger finger in Part I, before expanding that examination in Part II to consider diffuse causes of the condition. Both standard and cutting edge therapies are explained and explored.

The point is well made that we take our hands for granted until they don't work. I found the case studies especially compelling, and agree that the anecdotal evidence suggesting a link to vocation or avocation is strong. Given the heavy use of smartphones in our society, I found myself wondering if instances of trigger thumb will continue to rise, with a direct link to texting.

Joshua experienced two episodes of trigger finger, and used that experience to write a well-conceived and executed examination of the condition. That's a "take away" I can genuinely applaud. Most people would just complain about the problem. Joshua researched the syndrome, found an answer, and then shared the information.

The result is a thoughtful and useful compendium of practical data on a "simple" condition that isn't "simple" at all. I'm sorry I glazed over when I first heard about this book, but I'm not sorry that I read it, and you won't be either. Thorough, readable, and interesting, Joshua shows that by having the right information, you can make the right choices.

The "standard" treatment for trigger finger is, in theory, surgery. When you're done reading this book, I think you'll agree that surgery should be the option of last resort. The best medical decisions are based on informed consent, another point strongly made in this text. Joshua sets out to accomplish just that, inform the reader. The result is a resounding success.

Rana K. Williamson, PhD

INTRODUCTION

Introduction

It Snapped Suddenly

In the spring of 2007, while I was working on the computer, something strange happened with my right hand. I could make a fist, but when I released my fingers, the ring finger remained bent. I couldn't make it go up, or down. When it finally returned to an upright position on its own, it snapped upwards suddenly and painfully.

I had no idea what was going on, and frankly, I was scared. For 30 years, I stretched my small hands to play classical music at the piano. For more than 20 years, I taught piano. Now, as an online entrepreneur, I was working online. It was an understatement to say that I needed my hands to function normally!

For several days, I did nothing, hoping the condition would go away. I noticed a lot of clicking in the finger when it moved, and the incidents of "locking up" continued. I tried a splint from the drugstore, but it didn't help. I did notice a slight bump at the base of my ring finger and wondered if it was related to the problem. In the end, I gave in and went to our family orthopedist. He told me I had trigger finger. I'd never heard of the condition until that day.

The doctor discussed a potential steroid injection, but said the effect might only be temporary, and that it could return. Surgery was the best option. Using a wall chart, he explained that the issue was at the base of the finger where an incision would be made and the restricting elements released. The procedure would be performed in a hospital setting, but it would require just 15 minutes, and only a local anesthetic would be used.

Not knowing any more about the condition, and trusting his advice, I scheduled the procedure. Then I went home and started thinking about it. For me, personally, going straight to hand surgery didn't feel like the right option. There had to be another way. I started researching trigger finger.

One of the things that most interested me from the beginning was the possible connection between trigger finger and gout. I had also been experiencing pain in my large right toe, and I understood that gout stemmed from an excess of uric acid in the body. I knew enough about nutrition to realize my diet contained far too much sugar and fat for my own good.

Over the next few weeks, I repeatedly submerged my hand in warm water and massaged the area where the doctor had explained the incision would be made. I forced myself to do hand exercises, even if it was nothing more than wiggling my fingers to increase the range of motion. As the days passed, the clicking stopped, and the finger returned to normal.

One month later, however, the same thing happened to the ring finger on my left hand. Rather than go to the doctor again, I repeated the same heat, massage, and exercise techniques, and once again, successfully healed the condition. By then, I had learned that trigger finger happens most often in postmenopausal women. There is some controversy about whether or not certain jobs or activities increase the risk of developing the condition. I knew I'd abused my hands for years to master complicated musical passages, and I wondered if unknowingly I'd done this to myself.

Throughout my experience, I wanted to understand the cause of my trigger finger, and not to opt for a treatment that would either make me susceptible to a recurrence of the condition or worsen my existing symptoms.

I wanted to understand why this was happening to me. As a result, I discovered that there was nothing perplexing about this condition, which can be linked to numerous causal factors. Some are purely mechanical, but trigger finger can also present as a symptom of a larger disease, or it can even be a consequence of diet.

Although my trigger finger has not returned, I have compiled and updated my research to help others dealing not only with alleviating the conditions, but truly understanding why it happened in the first place.

PART I
TRIGGER FINGER EXPLAINED

Part I
Trigger Finger Explained

In the simplest terms, a trigger finger occurs when one or more fingers of the hand "stick" or become permanently bent toward the palm.

To understand this more clearly, hold out your hand and extend your thumb and forefinger the way you may have done when you were a child pretending to shoot an imaginary gun. Pull the "trigger," and you'll immediately understand what this condition looks like.

Trigger fingers fall into two major classes:

"Classic" trigger finger associated with specific trauma, dysfunction, or nodule growth at the base of the finger or thumb.

"Diffuse" trigger fingers that are symptoms of a larger "systemic" (system wide) problem, for instance, diabetes or gout.

We'll look at the difference between classic and diffuse trigger fingers more closely in Part II. For our purposes at the moment, "classic" trigger finger, in order of most common occurrence, affects:

- the ring,
- thumb,
- long,
- index,
- And little fingers.

Typically, trigger finger presents on the dominant hand, with one or more fingers and/or the thumb involved. Paradoxically, children under the age of six, and postmenopausal women age 40-60 are the most likely candidates to develop this problem.

How common is the Condition?

Over the past five years, medical science has revised its understanding of trigger finger. The condition was once thought to be exclusively a symptom of osteoarthritis. Certainly, people suffering from debilitating arthritis are prone to experiencing locked fingers, but they are not the primary sufferers of "classic" trigger finger syndrome.

Ergonomic and repetitive stress (cumulative trauma) disorders are the fastest growing category of work-related injuries in the United States and around the world. Many of these conditions affect the hands, including, but not limited to:

Epicondylitis, which is more commonly known as tennis elbow. It is characterized by pain from the elbow, radiating down the forearm, and into the wrist.

Tendonitis, which can occur in any location where the tendons become inflamed at their point of insertion to the bone.

Carpal tunnel syndrome, which causes pain in the hand and fingers due to the compression of a major nerve passing through the wrist.

De Quervain's Disease, also known as washerwoman's sprain, which is caused by inflammation of the tendon attached to the thumb, causing pain that radiates upwards into the lower arm.

And now, trigger finger.

With a new understanding of trigger finger as a repetitive stress injury, locked fingers directly attributable to inflammation and swelling of the tendons and ligaments at the base of the affected digit are now handled as specific-condition cases. They are no longer lumped in with locked fingers that are a secondary symptom of other conditions, and thus in need of different forms of treatment.

As repetitive stress injuries continue to increase in number, trigger finger has become a common ailment. Prior to the 1990s, however, it was relatively rare, and usually linked to direct physical trauma.

Who Gets It and Why?

According to the existing research, occupation does not have a bearing on the presentation of trigger finger. However, a growing body of anecdotal evidence suggests otherwise. Workers in almost any industry who rely on the repetitive movements of their thumb and finger, or who routinely grasp tools or objects with some degree of force, are at risk to experience this condition.

Musicians are a good example, as are long-haul truckers who grip the steering wheel for long periods of time and also experience the long-term effects of extended vibration. Rock climbers who use their fingers to secure themselves on steep, dangerous surfaces are at high risk, but even smokers can experience trigger thumb from years of using a lighter.

Different Types of Trigger Finger

Classic trigger finger symptoms present in a typical pattern and progress through predictable stages. However, fingers may become locked due to other causes, which will be discussed later in the body of this work.

"Classic" trigger finger is caused by an aberration in the functioning of the tendons specifically associated with the A1 pulley structure in the hand.

It is not difficult to locate these pulleys. Turn your hand over and look at your index finger. The A1 pulley is located just under the last crease of the finger where the digit joins the palm. The A2 is located above that crease, the A3 at the next crease toward the tip of the finger, and the A4 is above that crease.

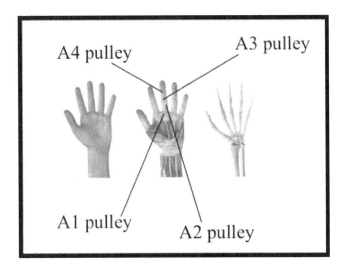

The proper name for the disorder affecting the A1 pulley is *stenosing tenosynovitis*. Unique characteristics of the condition include factors relative to:

Direction of movement - Some people will experience greater discomfort when their finger moves downward, while others find the upward motion the most painful. In some cases, when the bent finger releases, it is accompanied by a sharp, snapping motion. Other sufferers experience a slow, uncontrollable upward release.

Digits affected - Although most likely to occur in the thumb and forefinger of the dominant hand, trigger finger also affects the ring finger, and, in some cases, multiple fingers on one or both hands.

Case Study: Musician with Multiple Trigger Fingers

In 2010, in an article published in the Archives of Iranian Medicine, the authors reported a rare case of trigger finger in a 46-year-old, male musician. He was initially treated with two rounds of localized steroid injections for five trigger fingers on his left hand, and one on his right, but without significant relief.

The patient typically played guitar three hours a day, with even more time spent on his instrument on weekends. All of the involved fingers were used in his playing. There were no nodules clearly evident at the base of his fingers, but he could not make a fist, experiencing both pain and locked digits when he tried.

After a complete workup, doctors found no sign of thyroid abnormality, renal disease, gout, diabetes, or rheumatoid arthritis -- all conditions that can exhibit trigger finger as a secondary symptom.

Surgical release techniques were used on all the affected fingers. Only minimal post-surgical dressings were applied, and the man was encouraged to move the hand freely, but not to play his guitar for one month.

After 30 days passed, the musician returned to his job playing the guitar. He experienced no discomfort, and no locking of the formerly affected digits.

In 1998, a study published in the Journal of Hand Surgery (Trezies, et al) examined 178 patients and found no correlation between occupation and instances of trigger finger.

Long-standing wisdom has held that any job requiring the exertion of pressure in the palm while gripping forcefully would increase the risk of developing trigger finger. However, this case clearly illustrates that such force is not an absolute requirement for trigger finger to develop, and that an occupation can cause and/or intensify one or more locked fingers.

Source: Yavari, Masoud, Seyed Esmail Hassapour, and Seyed Mehdi Mosavizadeh. "Multiple Trigger Fingers in a Musician: A Case Report." Archives of Iranian Medicine, 2010 (13) 3: 251-252.

Differentiating the Condition from Arthritis

The term "trigger finger" is also used to describe the permanently bent fingers that are a consequence of severe osteoarthritis of the hand. While the appearance is much the same, the causes are completely different.

In arthritic cases, the joints lock in a bent position because of the degenerative nature of the condition. Arthritis erodes the cushioning materials in the joints, creating a painful "bone on bone" grinding.

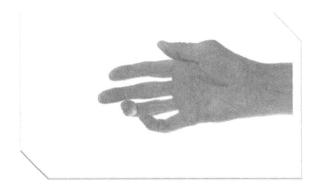

Over time, the tendons also deteriorate, and the fingers drop and often twist. In this case, however, the damaged tendons are not the primary cause of the locked fingers, but a progressive stage of a larger disease.

Arthritis sufferers can get some relief with therapy, pain medication (including corticosteroid injections), and assistive devices like splints. Once their joints lock, however, the deformity of their hands is permanent.

Classic trigger finger can be treated successfully by a variety of methods, although surgery may be required to resolve the condition permanently.

The Basic Mechanics of Classic Trigger Finger

Fibrous tendons connect muscles in the forearm to the bones of the fingers and thumb. The bones and muscles work together to allow the fingers to bend and to extend. Put your hand around your lower forearm or wrist, and open and close your fist several times. You'll be able to feel the muscles moving

Bands of arched ligaments on the surface of the bone hold the connective tendons in place to stabilize the interaction of the muscles and bones. These ligaments form a protective sheath. Normally, the tendons glide smoothly through the resulting "tunnel," which contains lubricating synovial fluid.

Anything that interrupts the tendons' ease of motion can lead to trigger finger. This may be caused by inflammation of the tendon itself, which, in turn, causes swelling. The tendon is then too large for the available space, and motion degrades. However, the problem can also originate in the ligaments, which may thicken, and obstruct the passage of the tendon.

Regardless of the cause, however, when the tendon cannot pass freely through the sheath, it pops or snaps as it pulls against the restrictions bearing down on it. When the available space for motion is sufficiently diminished, the tendon will no longer be able to move at all. At that point, the affected finger gets stuck in the "trigger" position.

(It's common to think of the affected finger being stuck in the "down" position, but it is also possible for the digit to be stuck "up," meaning the patient cannot bend the finger toward the palm.)

Fig. 1
Conditions Associated with Locked Digits

alcoholism

carpal tunnel
syndrome

diabetes

epilepsy

renal disease

smoking

amyloidosis

De Quervain's Disease

Dupuytren's
Contracture

gout

rheumatoid arthritis

thryoid abnormalities

tuberculosis

Progressive Symptoms

In classic cases of trigger finger, the symptoms progress along a predictable arc. The initial onset is subtle, and in almost all cases is ignored.

Morning Stiffness

The individual may first notice stiffness in the finger early in the morning. They may feel the need to make their hand "wake up" or "warm up." Generally this involves extending and stretching the fingers, which some people call "getting the blood to flow." Most trigger finger sufferers say they believed the stiffness to be an early sign of arthritis, which they dismissed as a normal part of aging.

Popping and Clicking

Once morning stiffness has presented, it won't be long before the finger begins to pop and click when moved. These sensations may be "felt" in the beginning, but over time they become audible, and may even be considered loud.

A Tender Nodule

When a trigger finger becomes noisy, tenderness at the base of the finger is inevitable. A small bump or nodule will appear at the *base* of the finger. This will be present just below the finger's bottom crease and slightly into the palm. (If you have a bump or nodule farther into the palm, you may be suffering from Dupuytren's Contracture, not classic trigger finger.)

A Word about Dupuytren's Contracture

The growth of small, benign lumps in the connective tissue of the *palm* of the hand can cause the tissues to contract, also drawing the fingers in toward the palm. These growths, however, are much closer to the center of the palm, near the largest crease, not at the base of the affected finger.

Dupuytren's Contracture presents slowly. The symptoms are initially mild, and there is no associated pain. This condition is not the same as trigger finger caused by tendon inflammation.

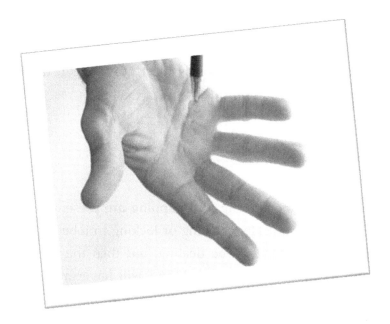

The cause of Dupuytren's Contracture is not known, although it appears to be hereditary, and is often associated with diabetes and epilepsy. People who drink and smoke heavily are also prone to the condition.

In severe cases, surgery is used to cut or to remove the affected tissues, thus releasing the tension. The recurrence rate after surgery is 50%. Consequently, some cases of Dupuytren's Contracture are now treated with direct injections of clostridium histolyticum, an enzyme which helps to break up the contracture.

Dupuytren's Contracture is fairly common, and it affects both genders, but is seen most often in men between the ages of 30 and 40. The condition is most prevalent in the United States, Canada, and Europe.

Catching and Locking

By the time clicking and popping are present, the finger will start periodically catching or locking in a bent condition. At first the effect will be fleeting, but then the sufferer will wake up with the finger bent, and will have great difficulty getting it to release. At this point, the swollen tendon is literally stuck inside its protective sheath. When it does manage to clear the space, it pops back in place suddenly and painfully.

Permanent Deformity

Soon, common everyday movements will cause the finger to lock up. The digit will remain in that position for hours, then days, and then it will not move at all. Typically this occurs when you reach to pick up an object. When you release your grip, the finger remains bent.

Most people try to massage the finger, or soak it in warm water to get it to turn loose, but unless these methods are used as a set program of therapy, they will become less and less effective over time until finally the finger stays bent toward the palm permanently.

Generally, it is at this point that the sufferer seeks medical attention. The bent finger has become a day-to-day liability, hindering the completion of common tasks.

Classifying the Stages of Trigger Finger

In the vast majority of cases, trigger finger comes on without warning. Patients may be able to look back and realize they were progressing through the symptoms, but at the time they ignored what was happening because it wasn't interfering with their lives.

There are four stages or "grades" of trigger finger:

Grade 1: The finger is stiff, usually in the morning, and the base may be tender, with a bump or nodule present just where the palm of the hand starts.

Grade 2: The motion of the fingers becomes uneven, with brief episodes of "triggering" or locking that release by themselves.

Grade 3: The affected finger will lock, but can only be released by manipulation and external force. Often the release is sudden and painful.

Grade 4: The deformity of the finger is pronounced and fixed, affecting the person's ability to use their hand and to perform everyday tasks.

The Quinnell Scale defines the progression in five stages:

Type 0 - Normal Movement
Type 1 - Uneven Movement
Type 2 - Actively Correctable
Type 3 - Passively Correctable
Type 4 - Fixed Deformity

Diagnosis of Trigger Finger

No specific tests are required to diagnose trigger finger. Some doctors prefer to have X-rays taken to rule out the presence of an injury. In general, however, diagnosis is based on a physical examination of the affected hand by a physician.

An oral history is taken, with the bulk of the diagnosis coming from a description of the symptoms experienced along with a consideration of occupation, and other activities that might contribute to repetitive stress.

If there is a visual or palpable nodule at the base of the finger, a diagnosis of classic trigger finger is all but assured. Some doctors will listen to the affected digit to confirm the presence of clicking and popping.

Trigger finger first entered the medical literature as an identifiable condition in 1850. Dr. A. Notta, an "interné" in Paris, published a description in the Archives Générales de Médecine, describing four adult patients age 20-60 with nodules on the flexor tendon of a finger that inhibited movement. Even today, these nodules are frequently referred to as "Notta's nodules."

If none of these symptoms are present, however, and the patient has a locked digit, then tests will be performed to rule out other conditions that have trigger finger as a secondary symptom. These include diabetes, gout, and rheumatoid arthritis, among others.

PART II
UNDERSTANDING TRIGGER FINGER
THE NEXT LEVEL

Part II

Understanding Trigger Finger; The Next Level

Current medical wisdom holds that surgery is the most effective treatment to release a trigger finger. Because no one is willing -- or should be willing -- to "go under the knife" unless it's absolutely necessary, most patients who see a doctor immediately want to know more about the condition before proceeding.

Exploring Specific Causes

The human hand is a wonderfully complex and dexterous creation that we tend to take for granted until it doesn't work properly. Basically, the mechanisms involved in the development of trigger finger can be likened to a pulley that isn't working properly. In fact, the first ligament at the base of the finger, the "A1 pulley" is normally the culprit in instances of locked fingers.

This ligament sits in a highly exposed position, just above the spot where people who work with their hands tend to develop calluses on their palms. The A1 absorbs the brunt of the pressure when the hand grips an object. Over time, the ligament tends to thicken in response, which blocks the opening of the tendon sheath. This makes it difficult for the tendon to slide back and forth through the opening and function properly.

When you bend your finger or thumb toward the palm of your hand, the tendon slides downward in the sheath and toward the arm. Straightening the thumb or finger pulls the tendon back out of the sheath and into the finger.

Getting the tendon past the swollen ligament may cause a sudden "popping" upward of the finger, something like the quick release when a jammed object is set free. Once this sudden release motion begins to occur, conditions inside the finger will get worse according to one of three predictable progressions.

The constricted action on the tendon will cause constant friction, which in turn will make the tendon swell. This compounds an existing bad situation, since the thickened ligament has already narrowed the opening of the tendon sheath.

The irritation from the tendon migrates to the lining of the sheath itself, which became inflamed and even narrower. Now, rather than constriction at the opening of the sheath, the entire passage is affected. The tissue at the opening of the sheath (base of the finger) becomes irritated, forming a small nodule or lump, which now creates an additional obstacle over which the tendon must pass.

Normally, the nodules that form are larger on the end toward the palm, and narrower toward the tendon sheath. This structure makes it very easy for the nodule to block the opening of the sheath and to become stuck. Think of the action as literally putting a cork in a bottle.

The self-perpetuating cycle of friction, inflammation, and swelling creates a perfect cascade of symptoms that ultimately narrow the sheath, or lead to its blockage so effectively, the tendon can no longer move. At this point, the condition is a "fixed deformity."

Diffuse Trigger Fingers

These factors, however, tend to exclusively describe classic trigger finger or nodular tenosynovitis. Diffuse tenosynovitis, which may be a symptom of a larger illness affecting the whole body, may not present the same way.

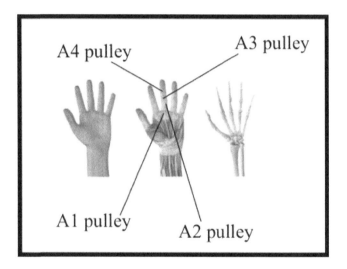

With classic trigger finger, the A1 pulley at the base of the finger is always involved, causing the finger to drop toward the palm of the hand. Trigger fingers that present from other locations, for instance the A2 pulley which is located in the pad of the finger below the second joint, may cause only a partial drop. It's even possible for just the top of the finger to be abnormally bent.

Given this distinction, it's important to understand all the other factors that may lead a finger joint to lock, deforming one or more digits on either hand.

The Role of the Synovium in Trigger Finger

Joints are surrounded by a membrane called the synovium, which produces a lubricating substance called synovial fluid. In consistency, this fluid is roughly as thick as a raw egg white. Normally, synovial fluid contains glucose, protein, and a few white and red blood cells. It is straw colored to clear, and moderately viscous, meaning it will bead up if dripped.

As a non-Newtonian fluid, however, the viscosity, or thickness of synovial fluid is subject to change from a variety of factors including, but not limited to.

Dehydration - As the body becomes dehydrated, it temporarily shuts down capillaries to divert the flow of blood to the brain and vital organs. The tissues deprived of their normal blood supply become clogged with cellular waste. The joints are one of the first areas affected, with pain and discomfort resulting.

Infection and inflammation - Initially inflammation may cause the synovial fluid to be less viscous or thinner, but in cases where a larger contributing illness is present, the opposite may occur. Rheumatoid arthritis (RA) is an autoimmune disease, which causes joint swelling and pain by attacking the synovial fluid and degrading its lubricating properties, leading to severe joint damage over time.

The presence or absence of chemicals in the synovial fluid contributes markedly to joint function. Testing this fluid may be part of the protocol of assessing non-typical trigger finger cases. These tests will not only look for bacterial infections, but also for high glucose levels associated with diabetes, lactate dehydrogenase present with RA, and uric acid crystals indicating gout.

Case Study: Bilateral Trigger Finger in a 7-Year-Old Boy after a Viral Infection

A seven-year-old boy presented with a bilateral case of trigger finger ten days after seeing the physician for hip pain and a limp. The child had no fever, and there had been no instance of trauma.

Lab tests, however, revealed an elevated erythrocyte sedimentation rate (ESR), which indicates the presence of inflammation. When the trigger finger appeared on the ring finger of each hand, the physician suspected a systemic cause.

Antibiotics are not useful in the treatment of viruses, so rest and increased fluid intake was recommended. This conservative wait-and-see approach sought to circumvent the usual response to trigger finger, which is to go straight to surgical intervention.

Within a month, the boy's hands had returned to normal. Although an unusual case, parents should be aware that in otherwise inexplicable cases of trigger finger, viral infection should not be ruled out.

Source: Sharma, Pundrique R., et al. "Bilateral Trigger Finger in a 7-Year-Old After a Viral Infection: Case Report." *The Journal of Hand Surgery*, 2010 (35) 4: 1334-1335.

Common Risk Factors

Even though classic trigger finger is now regarded as a repetitive stress injury, the exact combination of factors that leads to its development are still not clearly understood.

Some repetitive tasks that could result in the development of trigger finger include, but are not limited to:

- texting
- typing
- playing a musical instrument
- playing video games
- gripping a steering wheel for long periods
- the use of power tools
- the use of hand tools
- intense needlework (knitting, crocheting, and others)
- sport climbing, especially rock climbing

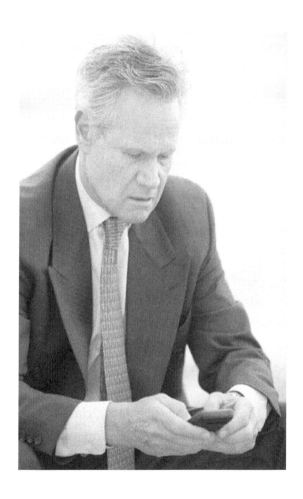

Other clear risk factors include:

Gender – Women are six times more likely than men to experience trigger finger.

Age – The condition is common in children under six years of age, and in adults of more than 40 years. It is most prevalent in individuals in their 50s or 60s.

Trauma - The syndrome often results from trauma or injury to the base of the fingers or palm.

Case Study: Trigger Finger Due to Trauma and Infection

In this case, a 38-year-old woman had experienced painful triggering of the long finger on her left hand for two months. Her problems began when she punctured herself with a kitchen knife at the base of the affected finger while cutting vegetables that had been washed in plain tap water.

Because the triggering seemed "classic," she initially received two corticosteroid injections to release the affected digit. Although initially successful, in one week's time, the finger was once again bent.

When occupational therapy failed to help her condition, surgery was performed. Due to the abnormalities detected during surgery and an over-abundance of fluid at the base of the finger, tests were performed, which came back positive for *Mycobacterium kansaii.*

The patient was given Azithromycin, Ethambutol, and Rifampin by mouth. Her finger healed from the surgery, she regained full range of motion in the hand, and no triggering behavior has returned.

This was a highly unusual case of trigger finger. The authors of the study examined 434 articles and found no other case of the disorder attributed to mycobacterium, which apparently entered the woman's system from the tap water at the time of her kitchen-related knife wound.

Source: Mejia, Hector, Mark Ryzewicz, and Frank Scott. "Trigger Finger Due to Tenosynovitis From Mycobacterium Kansasii Infection in an Immunocompetent Patient." *Orthopedics*, 2007 (30) 12.

Conditions Associated with Trigger Finger

Some primary health issues may include trigger finger as a symptom or secondary effect.

Diabetes - Diabetics often experience locked fingers, which doctors attribute in their case to an overabundance of glucose in the blood.

Rheumatoid Arthritis - RA sufferers deal with inflamed and swollen joints on a regular basis. The hands are particularly susceptible to these issues, and thus to episodes of trigger finger.

Other conditions that often present with locked fingers include:

amyloidosis **-** A condition in which the protein amyloid is present in abnormally high levels in the internal organs, in particular, the liver.

gout **-** A painful inflammation of the joints, in particular the big toe, due to an over-abundance of uric acid in the body.

Carpal tunnel syndrome - A condition caused by repetitive stress in the wrist resulting in pain and tingling. Both carpal tunnel syndrome, and the surgery typically used to treat it, can cause trigger finger.

De Quervain's Disease – This disease causes pain in the wrist, and affects the tendons connected to the thumb.

Cases of underactive thyroid (hypothyroidism) and mucopolysaccharide storage disorders (rare, life-threatening metabolic conditions) may also cause instances of trigger finger. Many patients with tuberculosis experience locked digits, as do those who suffer from the inflammatory intestinal disorder, Crohn's Disease.

Congenital Trigger Thumb in Children

Triggering digits are fairly uncommon in children, and when they do occur, they appear in the thumb 86% of the time. Frequently the condition is caused by a thickening of the flexor tendon due to the presence of a typical Notta's nodule.

A third of the patients who exhibit this condition are from families with a history of the disorder. Of those, 20-30% are affected in both hands. In many cases, treatment is delayed until the first year of life has passed, since 30% of cases resolve spontaneously. If that does not occur, the routine surgical release of the A1 pulley is performed.

The triggering of the digits does not occur in the womb, but happens after birth. This condition is different from a congenital clasped thumb, which has the appearance of lying across the palm as if the child were about to close his fist over the digit and hold it. Some children are also born without the extensor pollicis longus, which is a forearm muscle that serves in part to stretch the thumb.

Both of these conditions require a completely different kind of treatment than classic trigger finger or thumb.

Is There a Cure? Treatment Options

The "cure" for trigger finger depends entirely on what kind of triggering is being addressed. For classic cases of trigger finger, the two dominant recommendations currently offered by medical science are steroid injections and/or surgery.

Many individuals, however, have been able to heal themselves with alternative techniques including heat and massage. Splinting may also be effective, including small splints that are used at night to keep the finger extended. With these methods, the dominant goal is softening the affected tendon to reduce swelling and inflammation.

Conventional Treatments for Trigger Finger

Because most patients wait to seek medical intervention for their trigger finger until the digit is more or less fixed and immobile, doctors tend to recommend two standard interventions: steroid injections and surgery.

Steroid Injections

In about 86% of cases, trigger finger can be resolved with two steroid injections. The process is not painful. A numbing solution, lidocaine, is applied to the area before the needle is inserted.

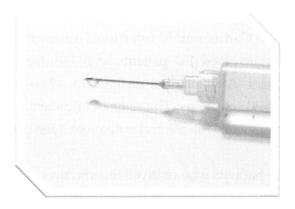

The injected cortisone is an anti-inflammatory, intended to reduce swelling, which can be present at multiple points in a classic case:

- the tendon itself,
- the tendon sheath,
- the ligaments, and
- the associated nodule.

Since any kind of swelling can cause a digit to lock, steroid injections may be effective regardless of the cause of the triggering. Typically, however, placement of the injection is at the base of the finger.

Because these injections are localized, there is no need to be concerned about side effects from the cortisone. Many patients prefer to try this non-invasive form of treatment.

Case Study: Corticosteroid Injection Treatment vs. Surgery
This study involved 137 patients with 150 digits affected by trigger finger. After random assignment, 49 patients received corticosteroid injections. The remaining patients were treated with percutaneous release and outpatient open surgery.

Of the patients who received the injection:

57% were cured with one shot,
86% were cured with two shots.

Remission or "cure" was achieved in 100% of the surgical treatments. Both the percutaneous and open surgery methods were found to be equally effective in relieving cases of trigger finger, and both were superior to corticosteroid injections.

Source: Sato, Edson S., Joao B. Gomes dos Santos, Joao C. Belloti, Walter M. Albertoni, and Flavio Faloppa. "Treatment of Trigger Finger: Randomized Clinical Trial Comparing the Methods of Corticosteroid Injection, Percutaneous Release, and Open Surgery." *Rheumatology Advance Access*, 2011 (10).

Surgical Intervention

There are two main types of surgery to repair trigger finger: percutaneous trigger finger release and open surgery.

Percutaneous Trigger Finger Release

In this procedure, the surgeon inserts a needle into the base of the affected finger and uses the implement to divide the affected A1 pulley. This serves to release the tendon, so it can once again slide smoothly through the tendon sheath.

Open Surgery

In open surgery, a small incision is made in the palm at the base of the affected finger. This gives the surgeon visual access to the A1 pulley, which is then divided to free up the action of the tendon. If a nodule is present, this form of surgery also allows the physician to more closely examine its structure and nature.

New Innovation: Endoscopic Surgery

Endoscopy is a relatively new technique to accomplish surgical trigger finger release. It provides the best of both "worlds." Like percutaneous surgery, endoscopy is less invasive, but because the endoscope is a small video camera, the surgeon can still visually inspect the area as he would with open surgery.

The incision from an endoscopic procedure is less than one-eighth to one-quarter of an inch in length, and no stitches are required, allowing for normal use of the hand almost immediately.

Non-Surgical and Alternative Treatments

Patients who opt for non-surgical intervention of trigger finger normally use a combination of immobilization via splinting, exercises, heat therapy, and massage.

Splinting

Although few doctors recommend using a splint to treat trigger finger, the method is a popular self-help solution, which may be effective in mild cases of the condition. Often the splint is worn at night, to keep the finger from being stiff and locking up first thing in the morning.

When used in combination with heat, massage, and NSAIDs (over-the-counter anti-inflammatory drugs like naproxen, ibuprofen, and diclofenac), splints should be worn for a minimum of six weeks.

Exercises

Not all patients who rely on exercise to relieve trigger finger follow a formal, prescribed routine. Opening and closing the fist, wiggling the fingers, and stretching to increase the flexibility of the palm are all recommended. The idea is to break up the constricting nodule, increase blood flow, and thin the tendon to ease its passage through the tendon sheath.

Some examples of possible exercises include:

__Palm Up Isolated Exercise__ - Hold your arm out, bent at the elbow, palm up. Make a fist and release your fingers, extending fully. This action strengthens the extensor muscles and stretches the flexor tendons. This will help to break down the adhesion at the base of the affected finger and also to thin the tendon so it moves more freely.

__Finger Stretches__ - Place your index and middle finger side by side in the extended position. Place the two fingers against the palm of your opposite hand. Using that hand, push the fingers back toward you, past full extension, rotating slightly until you feel a pulling sensation in your palm. Hold for 12 to 15 seconds and release. Repeat, rotating slightly away from you. Do the same for the middle and ring finger held together, and then the ring and little finger.

__Using Resistance__ - Trigger finger occurs often in people who grip object repeatedly. This action uses the flexor muscles. To exercise the extensor muscles, hold your hand up with fingers straight, then bend the fingers at the knuckles forming a 90-degree angle. Move the thumb inward and place it under and against the extended finger. Wrap a heavy rubber band around your fingers and thumb. Practice moving the fingers upward against the resistance of the band.

Heat

The goal of heat therapy with trigger finger is to soften the affected areas, making them more subject to manipulation. Many practitioners advocate a combination of heat and cold. Heat is used to enhance massage and exercise options, while cold applications help to control inflammation and to relieve pain.

First Person Account - Wet Heat for Trigger Thumb

Several years ago, Alice experienced a painful trigger thumb. Her doctor recommended surgery, but she consulted her Rolfer before agreeing to the procedure. (Rolfing is a technique that works to achieve vertical body realignment through deep muscle massage.) He suggested that she try applying wet heat to the affected thumb.

Alice put boiling water in a stainless steel travel mug. She suspended her thumb over the water without touching it, using the rest of her hand to seal the mug and keep the steam contained. Her goal was to soften the thumb joint. She repeated this process for 8-10 minutes at a time, four to five times a day.

Over a period of three days, the joint did soften, and ten years later, Alice had not experienced a return of the condition.

Source: My Dance with Cancer. "Trigger Finger Trigger Thumb Cured via Simple Solution." phkillscancer.com. http://phkillscancer.com/natural-treatment/trigger-finger-trigger-thumb-cured-via-simple-solution (Accessed March 2013.

Massage

The goal of self-massaging a digit affected by trigger finger is to enhance the flow of blood to the area. This will help to lubricate the joint. Hold your finger in a comfortable position and use a circular motion to rub across the joint for 2-3 minutes. Use this simple technique in concert with exercise and heat and/or cold therapies.

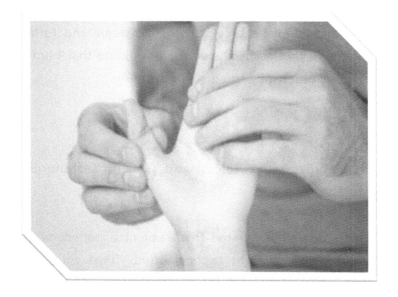

The Chiropractic Approach to Trigger Finger

Chiropractors emphasize reducing the contracture of the trigger finger by stretching the tendons and muscles in combination with ice and heat therapies. Many also recommend acupuncture at the site, and running along the line of the tendon from origin to insertion. This helps to release tension and strain on the tendon, and, if a nodule is present, to lessen its entrapment.

Both the Active Release Technique (ART) and the Graston Technique are also used. ART is movement-based, soft tissue manipulation to treat adhesions and scar tissue in overused muscles. The Graston Technique is instrument-assisted soft tissue manipulation to break down scar tissue and to lessen restrictions in the fascia, the connective tissue that binds the muscles and other soft structures of the body.

Case Study: Active Release and Graston Techniques for Trigger Thumb

This study followed the treatment of a patient with an unresolved case of right trigger thumb. Two chiropractic-based therapies were used, the Active Release Technique, and the Graston Technique. The goal was to rebuild thumb extensor strength. Ice was used to control pain and inflammation.

Eight treatments were administered, with the patient showing improved range of motion, a lessening of pain, and better function. The patient also expressed personal satisfaction with the outcome of the conservative treatment approach.

Conventional treatments of this condition involve either corticosteroid injections or the surgical removal of imposing tissue. Soft tissue manipulation, however, is a non-invasive approach with results at least equal to, and perhaps better than, the accepted treatment norms.

According to research cited in the study, corticosteroid injections are effective within two weeks, but wear off in three months. Surgery offers a 91% success rate, but many patients do not want to have the procedure.

In patients with carpal tunnel syndrome, ART therapy alone has shown a 71 % success rate. The authors of this study concluded that based on their success with a single patient, soft-tissue-based therapies for trigger thumb are worthy of greater investigation.

Source: Howitt, Scott, Jerome Wing, and Sonja Zbukovec. "The Conservative Treatment of Trigger Thumb Using Graston Techniques and Active Release Techniques." *Journal of the Canadian Chiropractic Association*, 2006 (50) 4: 249-254.

Acupuncture and Trigger Finger

All too often, conventional medicine regards acupuncture as a viable therapy option for chronic pain, while failing to recognize its potential efficacy in resolving specific problems in the first place. Trigger finger may well be one of those issues.

Consider the case of a 50-year-old woman, whose story was written up in *Medical Acupuncture: A Journal for Physicians by Physicians*, by Rowena Archibald, MD. ("Treatment of a Case of Post-Traumatic Neuralgia, Vol. 13:10) In 1999, the woman complained of a burning sensation in her right middle finger, with severe pain extending into the palm, and a heightened sensitivity to cold.

In 1996, she had surgery for trigger finger in that digit and required a second surgery in 1997. The second surgery revealed a neuroma in the damaged area. Through two additional surgeries to address the nerve damage, the patient's pain grew increasingly worse. In addition, the woman suffered from both fibromyalgia and rheumatoid arthritis.

Only after four surgeries was it suggested that she try acupuncture, and then only to control her chronic pain. After four months of treatment, she reported that her pain had decreased by half.

One can only wonder what acupuncture might have done for her in the first place, going all the way back to when the original trigger finger presented.

In a case study ("Trigger Finger in a Male with Diabetes Successfully Treated with Acupuncture and Osteopathic Manipulative Treatment") by Robert Schulman, Aleksandr

Levchenko, and Sergio R. Lombardo published in *Medical Acupuncture* (February 2013), the patient was treated once a week for eight weeks with osteopathic manipulation including:

- myofascial release,
- muscle energy,
- manipulation and articulation of the carpal bones.

These targeted massage techniques were paired with acupuncture. The man exhibited significant improvement, and a year later showed no symptoms.

The main goal of acupuncture treatment is to balance "energy" in the body along pathways defined by traditional Eastern medicine. In the case of the woman treated after four surgical procedures, she not only experienced diminished pain, but improved appearance of her scars, with a lessening of redness and inflammation.

Although acupuncture is not typically recommended for trigger finger, there is evidence to suggest that as a compliment to treatments like massage and the application of heat and cold, it could be useful, especially in reducing inflammation in the affected digit.

Where to Get Help

Most people who suffer from trigger finger initially consult with their family physician. A general practitioner is perfectly capable of diagnosing a classic case of trigger finger. Expect to receive a recommendation for corticosteroid injections or surgery, and likely a referral to an orthopedic surgeon or a hand specialist.

If, however, you are not suffering from a classic trigger finger, but rather a locked digit associated with another condition, these solutions will offer only temporary relief. Never move forward with a medical procedure of any kind, until you are completely comfortable with the diagnosis you have received.

A trigger finger can be the sign of a larger problem, and should not be dismissed as a simple malfunction of the A1 pulley in the finger.

Latest Research

The mechanics of classic trigger finger are well understood. When the condition presents as an aspect of a broader, systemic disorder, however, treatment is more individualized, and must be dealt with in the context of the unique particulars.

The most recent research has focused on better diagnostic techniques paired with an improved placement of corticosteroid injections. Typically, imaging tests have not been used in cases of trigger finger if, for no other reason than that the tests are expensive.

Given the rising cost of health care and health insurance in the United States, doctors have not usually regarded ultrasound as a necessary medical expense for something so "simple" as trigger finger. At the same time, however, there is a growing emphasis on less invasive medicine, and a high degree of surgical fear on the part of the general populace.

The presence of drug-resistant bacteria in U.S. hospitals in recent years, beginning with methicillin-resistant staphylococcus aureus (MRSA) and progressing to the most recent carbapenem-resistant enterobacteriaceae (CRE) outbreaks have many patients rightfully wary of any kind of surgical treatment -- including the resolution of a "simple" trigger finger.

In the standard course of a trigger finger diagnosis, doctors rely on physical examination, the taking of an oral history, and occasionally X-rays. They then recommend corticosteroid injections or surgery, with the emphasis being on surgery, which has a history of a 90% success rate. Recent research with image-guided administration of corticosteroids suggests, however, that the same level of success can be achieved with one injection.

In 2008, research published by the *American Institute of Ultrasound in Medicine* showed that sonography can allow direct visualization of the A1 pulley structure in the hand. When physicians can judge what is happening in the hand without a surgical incision, they can better target the placement of corticosteroid injections, thus increasing their effectiveness.

In 2009, a second study outlined an ultrasound-guided A1 pulley injection technique showing a one-year success rate of 90% as compared to 56-57% with blind injections. (It should be noted that while the authors of this study accepted the blind injection statistics recorded in a study by Peters-Veluthamaningal, et al, in 2008, there are numerous studies in the literature involving injections, all with conflicting estimates of efficacy.)

The guided injection method targets a triangle under the A1 pulley bordered by the FDS and FDP tendons, the velar plate, the distal metacarpal bone, and the pulley itself.

By using fine needles, and a low dose of corticosteroid, the team achieved a 94% success rate at six months, falling to 90% at one year (with no instances of pierced tendons, a frequent consequence of blind injections.) For recurrent cases of trigger finger, the researchers planned to develop an ultrasound-guided proximal A1 pulley release technique.

While the traditional surgery is still widely recommended by physicians, there is ample evidence to illustrate that less invasive, more conservative treatments are as effective. Patients who are aware of the advances in sonography should discuss guided injections with their physician before opting for surgery.

With injections already returning the potential for as high as an 86% success rate (according to some case studies), fine tuning their administration could make corticosteroid therapy the preferred option over surgery.

PART III
CONCLUDING REMARKS

Part III

Concluding Remarks

In the introduction, I described the onset of my experiences with trigger finger, one with the ring finger of each hand, beginning with my dominant right hand. I mentioned that from the beginning, I was intrigued by the potential connection between locked digits and gout. After researching trigger finger in depth, I am even more convinced that diet plays a role in creating a susceptibility to this condition.

As I quickly discovered, it's not hard to track down a self-perpetuating cascade of factors that conspire to make Americans some of the unhealthiest, most overweight people on this planet. Consequently, we're suffering from all kinds of health problems that stem directly from what we're eating.

Dietary Factors and Trigger Finger

Over the past five years, increasing attention has been paid to the poor quality of the American diet and the resulting epidemic of obesity in this country. Fully two-thirds of all adults in the United States are overweight, and 1 in 3 children battle weight issues. Two conditions associated with obesity that also are tied to episodes of trigger finger are gout and diabetes.

Termed an "arthritic" condition, gout occurs when uric acid builds up in the joints, causing sudden and extreme pain, with accompanying redness and swelling. Although most often associated with the big toe, gout also affects the feet, ankles, knees, wrists, and hands.

Type 2 diabetes is caused by high levels of sugar in the blood. Diabetics are particularly prone to trigger finger because they also experience "diabetic hand syndrome." The symptoms include skin thickening, and limited range of motion in the joints. It is quite common for people with gout to also be type 2 diabetics.

Diet has come to the forefront of the health care debate in the United States because so many conditions, including type 2 diabetes, can be completely cured by healthy eating and weight loss. A major culprit in the thickening of the American waistline is high fructose corn syrup (HFCS), which is the primary source of calories in the U.S. today. HFCS is in virtually everything from soft drinks (especially diet drinks) to hot dog buns.

One of the known side effects of fructose is the elevation of uric acid in the human body. This, in turn, leads to chronic, low-level inflammation, which in turn leads to obesity, cardiovascular disease, hypertension, stroke, kidney disease, cancer, vertigo, and gout.

As if that cycle were not sufficiently vicious, the average consumer of diet drinks has three a day. Consuming just one diet drink a day raises a woman's chance of developing type 2 diabetes by 33 percent. These drinks are also packed with sodium, which makes you thirsty. Drink one, and you want another, but diet soda will never satisfy your thirst. It will, however, systematically pump more and more fructose into your system.

Take this matter of thirst a step farther. Sodas do not satisfy a human's need for water. Chronic dehydration is widespread in America, effecting just about everyone. As the body dehydrates, the joints feel the effect first, leading to a thickening of the synovium, the production of less lubricating synovial fluid, and thus decreased range of motion and pain.

Chronic dehydration also causes low energy and fatigue, constipation and other digestive disorders, high and low blood pressure, respiratory issues, weight gain, and the acidification of the system. Too much acid in the system can lead to urinary dysfunction . . . which leads to the build-up of uric acid . . . which leads to gout . . . and puts us right back where we started.

While we cannot say, "If you eat this, you will develop trigger finger," we can say that the American diet puts us all at risk for a wide range of health issues, including joint dysfunction -- and thus, trigger finger.

A Broader Problem

With any case of trigger finger, however, it's important to realize that you may be dealing with a primary condition relative to a malfunctioning ligament-tendon "partnership," or you may be looking at the symptom of a larger, systemic problem. I had never heard of trigger finger until my ring finger locked up, and I certainly had no idea about "diffuse" trigger fingers until I began this project.

Although at the time, the doctor did not tell me that my locked finger was the result of a repetitive stress injury, I intuitively assumed I had stressed my hands from years of playing the piano. Like most people who present with a "classic" trigger finger, I assumed my age and the early onset of arthritis were factors.

Consequently, I was presented with classic options -- steroid injections or surgery. Had I known what I know now, I might have chosen to try the injections, as their efficacy is much better than was initially suggested to me, in my opinion. By the same token, I would probably be even less likely today to opt for surgery than I was then, for the simple reason that as a pianist, I didn't want anyone cutting on my hands.

I have had no recurrence of my trigger finger, but I am now more vigilant about exercising my hands in warm water, keeping myself hydrated, and staying away from the "standard" American diet in favor of a more plant-based way of eating. These are personal choices for me, but I do believe that my poor diet and life-long refusal to drink enough water had an adverse effect on my joints.

Many times in the literature I have read statements by doctors saying that treating a case of trigger finger conservatively with heat and massage is a palliative only and not a "fix." In my case, this has not proven to be true, and I see a great deal of wisdom in helping the body to heal itself by thinning the affected tendon with exercise, and softening the joint with heat and massage. Our joints will do what they are designed to do if we give them half a chance.

Although I frankly struggled to get through many of the case studies I read during my research, I learned that it's often a mistake to treat every trigger finger as "classic." In the body of the text, and in the summaries I've included at the end of the book, you'll find cases of trigger finger linked to the presence of benign masses, including fatty lipomas, and to bacterial infections with a similarity to tuberculosis.

One man suffered ten locked trigger fingers that were caused by a combination of a life-long struggle with poor circulation of the hands aggravated to a crisis point when he began to use vibrating power tools daily to earn his living. A guitarist with no painful nodules present still experienced five locked fingers that seemed directly attributed to the hours he spent playing.

The point I'm trying to make is that trigger finger is not a "one size fits all" problem, although it is frequently treated that way. Surgical release does offer a high success rate, but not everyone wants to go that route. It would be a mistake to dismiss more conservative forms of treatment when the literature plainly shows that with diligent attention, locked digits can be handled via other methods.

Chronic Inflammation in the Body

To me, the key factor is inflammation, which is critical in a host of modern diseases including cancer. Any method that controls the inflammation of the affected tendons and joints will improve, if not resolve trigger finger. This is my opinion, based on my personal experience and my research on the subject.

(For more information about the negative effects of chronic inflammation see: *Younger Next Year* by Chris Crowley and Henry S. Lodge, and this video presentation by Dr. Michael Greger, "Uprooting the Leading Causes of Death," at NurtritionFacts.org http://nutritionfacts.org/video/uprooting-the-leading-causes-of-death/)

In my research, I have also tried to understand the relationship between autoimmune diseases and episodes of trigger finger. It is clearly associated with diabetes, rheumatoid arthritis, and Crohn's Disease, but I have also seen links to both fibromyalgia and lupus. In all autoimmune diseases, the body's immune responses turn against the body itself. Prolonged inflammation is the consequence. I am not a medical doctor, but the list of autoimmune diseases runs to more than 150 conditions.

Fig. II
Autoimmune Diseases

Acute Disseminated Encephalomyelitis (ADEM)
Acute necrotizing hemorrhagic leukoencephalitis
Addison's disease
Agammaglobulinemia
Alopecia areata
Amyloidosis
Ankylosing spondylitis
Anti-GBM/Anti-TBM nephritis
Antiphospholipid syndrome (APS)
Autoimmune angioedema
Autoimmune aplastic anemia
Autoimmune dysautonomia
Autoimmune hepatitis
Autoimmune hyperlipidemia
Autoimmune immunodeficiency
Autoimmune inner ear disease (AIED)
Autoimmune myocarditis
Autoimmune oophoritis
Autoimmune pancreatitis
Autoimmune retinopathy

Autoimmune thrombocytopenic purpura (ATP)
Autoimmune thyroid disease
Autoimmune urticaria
Axonal & neuronal neuropathies
Balo disease
Behcet's disease
Bullous pemphigoid
Cardiomyopathy
Castleman disease
Celiac disease
Chagas disease
Chronic fatigue syndrome
Chronic inflammatory demyelinating polyneuropathy (CIDP) Chronic recurrent multifocal ostomyelitis (CRMO)
Churg-Strauss syndrome
Cicatricial pemphigoid/benign mucosal pemphigoid
Crohn's disease
Cogans syndrome
Cold agglutinin disease
Congenital heart block
Coxsackie myocarditis
CREST disease
Essential mixed cryoglobulinemia
Demyelinating neuropathies
Dermatitis herpetiformis
Dermatomyositis

Devic's disease (neuromyelitis optica)

Discoid lupus

Dressler's syndrome

Endometriosis

Eosinophilic esophagitis

Eosinophilic fasciitis

Erythema nodosum

Experimental allergic encephalomyelitis

Evans syndrome

Fibromyalgia

Fibrosing alveolitis

Giant cell arteritis (temporal arteritis)

Giant cell myocarditis

Glomerulonephritis

Goodpasture's syndrome

Granulomatosis with Polyangiitis (GPA) (formerly called Wegener's Granulomatosis)

Graves' disease

Guillain-Barre syndrome

Hashimoto's encephalitis

Hashimoto's thyroiditis

Hemolytic anemia

Henoch-Schonlein purpura

Herpes gestationis

Hypogammaglobulinemia

Idiopathic thrombocytopenic purpura (ITP)

IgA nephropathy

IgG4-related sclerosing disease

Immunoregulatory lipoproteins

Inclusion body myositis

Interstitial cystitis

Juvenile arthritis

Juvenile diabetes (Type 1 diabetes)

Juvenile myositis

Kawasaki syndrome

Lambert-Eaton syndrome

Leukocytoclastic vasculitis

Lichen planus

Lichen sclerosus

Ligneous conjunctivitis

Linear IgA disease (LAD)

Lupus (SLE)

Lyme disease, chronic

Meniere's disease

Microscopic polyangiitis

Mixed connective tissue disease (MCTD)

Mooren's ulcer

Mucha-Habermann disease

Multiple sclerosis

Myasthenia gravis

Myositis

Narcolepsy

Neuromyelitis optica (Devic's)

Neutropenia

Ocular cicatricial pemphigoid

Optic neuritis

Palindromic rheumatism

PANDAS (Pediatric Autoimmune Neuropsychiatric Disorders Associated with Streptococcus)

Paraneoplastic cerebellar degeneration

Paroxysmal nocturnal hemoglobinuria (PNH)

Parry Romberg syndrome

Parsonnage-Turner syndrome

Pars planitis (peripheral uveitis)

Pemphigus

Peripheral neuropathy

Perivenous encephalomyelitis

Pernicious anemia

POEMS syndrome

Polyarteritis nodosa

Type I, II, & III autoimmune polyglandular syndromes

Polymyalgia rheumatica

Polymyositis

Postmyocardial infarction syndrome

Postpericardiotomy syndrome

Progesterone dermatitis

Primary biliary cirrhosis

Primary sclerosing cholangitis

Psoriasis

Psoriatic arthritis

Idiopathic pulmonary fibrosis

Pyoderma gangrenosum

Pure red cell aplasia

Raynauds phenomenon

Reactive Arthritis

Reflex sympathetic dystrophy

Reiter's syndrome

Relapsing polychondritis

Restless legs syndrome

Retroperitoneal fibrosis

Rheumatic fever

Rheumatoid arthritis

Sarcoidosis

Schmidt syndrome

Scleritis

Scleroderma

Sjogren's syndrome

Sperm & testicular autoimmunity

Stiff person syndrome

Subacute bacterial endocarditis (SBE)

Susac's syndrome

Sympathetic ophthalmia

Takayasu's arteritis

Temporal arteritis/Giant cell arteritis

Thrombocytopenic purpura (TTP)

Tolosa-Hunt syndrome

Transverse myelitis

Type 1 diabetes

Ulcerative colitis

Undifferentiated connective tissue disease (UCTD)

Uveitis

Vasculitis

Vesiculobullous dermatosis

Vitiligo

Wegener's granulomatosis (now termed Granulomatosis with Polyangiitis (GPA)

You will certainly want to be evaluated by a competent medical professional, but make sure that you are giving your informed consent to any procedure to which you agree. That means, know all the facts, ask all the questions, and request all the tests. Until you are satisfied with your diagnosis, it's not a "done deal."

PART IV
MANAGING TRIGGER FINGER:
RESOURCES

Part IV
Managing Trigger Finger: Resources

While you are determining how to address your trigger finger from a therapeutic perspective, there will be issues of management, both psychological and physical.

Living with a Person with Trigger Finger

"Living" with trigger finger isn't like coping with a life-threatening illness. It's about understanding the mechanics not just of your hand, but of how you use your hands. Since my two episodes with the syndrome, for instance, I can't carry plastic grocery sacks the same way. My ring fingers are weaker, and if I strain them unduly they almost feel as if they're going to come out of socket. I have had to teach myself to shift the weight to protect those two fingers.

I have tried to research the statistics about incidence and recurrence of trigger finger, but have had little success. Trigger finger is most often lumped in with work-related injuries, so I don't know if I'm looking at numbers about carpal tunnel syndrome instead of the relevant data I want. Therefore, I feel that I am living with the aftermath of a condition that, if aggravated, could return.

If you or your loved one are experiencing trigger finger for the first time, there are some things to consider. Depending on your occupation, you may not be able to do your job. We completely take for granted that our fingers will work. Even if we think about the onset of arthritis, the idea is of some stiffness or aches and pains. Trigger finger is a bigger deal.

Trying to function with a bent finger was incredibly frustrating. Just getting dressed in the morning, going about my normal routine, washing dishes -- all were made harder. It wasn't just that it got in the way of my playing the piano, it got in the way of everything! We don't think about how we use our hands. We just do it. The bent finger didn't necessarily hurt if I hit it, but it was just in the way. I had to rethink every single thing I did.

You will be frustrated with yourself, and anyone who relies on you to do anything with your hands will likely be frustrated as well. It is this sense of impatience that leads people to go straight for the surgery. That's what I almost did, but now, knowing all that I know about the condition, I'm glad I didn't.

In the following section we'll look at some assistive devices that can make short-term management of trigger finger somewhat easier. Splints may help you to keep your finger straight, but it will still be awkward. There is no substitution for patience in dealing with trigger finger. Give yourself time to be comfortable with the treatment approach that seems to best fit your personal medical philosophy and lifestyle.

If that means alternative therapies like acupuncture, chiropractic techniques, massage, and heat treatments, a minimum of six weeks may pass before you see any results. If you opt for corticosteroid injections, you may see relief in under two weeks. For surgical variants, your recovery will likely be two weeks to a month for full healing. Regardless, there is time involved and we humans tend to be an impatient lot.

The most important thing is to try to understand, if possible, what caused your trigger finger to happen in the first place, and what, if anything in your life can be altered (including diet) to prevent a recurrence.

Relevant Websites

The Electronic Textbook of Hand Surgery
http://www.eatonhand.com/hw/hw022.htm

A well-illustrated site with videos providing an overview of trigger finger and potential treatments.

Trigger Finger: Definition, by the Mayo Clinic Staff
http://www.mayoclinic.com/health/trigger-finger/DS00155

The Mayo Clinic is one of the world's premier medical centers. Its website is a recognized compendium of easily accessible medical information.

Medscape Reference: Trigger Thumb
http://emedicine.medscape.com/article/1244815-overview

Comprehensive illustrated article on the onset, progression, and treatment of trigger thumb.

Surgery for the Release of Trigger Finger by Drs. Gutow and Schneider
http://www.youtube.com/watch?v=zSFUpNeAIBA&lr=1

A short video showing a trigger finger release surgery. (Please note that this video does contain graphic surgical content.)

YNN News Report on Trigger Finger
http://berkshires.ynn.com/content/health/509040/healthy-living--trigger-finger/

A video news article on the details of trigger finger.

Arthritis and Trigger Finger
http://www.webmd.com/osteoarthritis/guide/trigger-finger

A comprehensive article from WebMD on the basics of trigger finger including causes, symptoms, diagnosis, and treatments.

Trigger Finger

http://www.nhs.uk/conditions/Triggerfinger/Pages/Introd
uction.aspx

A UK article explaining causes and treatment of trigger
finger.

Trigger Finger Products

Splints

Trigger finger splints are normally small in profile,
generally fitting over the knuckle, with the goal of
straightening the finger to prevent popping and locking. They
are often worn at night. One of the more popular and
inexpensive models is made by:

Active Innovations
www.braceability.com/trigger-finger-splints-trigger-finger-
treatment

A more subtle approach, especially good for women, is
the wire E.D.S. Ring Splint:

www.edsringsplints.com/trigger-finger-splint.html

Heat and Cold Therapy

Choosing methods to deliver heat and cold treatment is purely a matter of personal choice. If you are using hot water and steam to create heat in an isolated environment, be especially cautious not to burn yourself. Moist heat works well, for instance a wet washcloth that has been warmed in the microwave.

You might also consider liniments or sports creams that generate heat. Many of these also have ingredients that return an analgesic effect.

Therapy Gloves

Meridian Glove
meridianglove.com

The Meridian Glove seeks to combine both hand alignment and magnet therapy. It purports to relieve pain associated with arthritis, repetitive strain injuries, tendonitis, trigger finger, and trigger thumb. The magnets are placed to correspond with meridians in the hand. The site explains meridians in this way, "Meridians are the channels that allow the universal life energy, also known as chi(ki), prana, or shakti to flow throughout the body. These rivers of pure energy nourish the internal organs and tissues with this healing energy. When the energy is blocked, pain and illness are the result."

Prolotex Far Infrared Therapy Gloves
www.horsemanshop.com/doc/3-fold-gloves.pdf

These gloves claim to help relieve joint and muscle pain, as well as pain and numbness from arthritis, Raynaud's Syndrome, carpal tunnel or repetitive motion syndrome, and trigger finger. According to the site, "PROLOTEX™ specially formulated bio-ceramic material, safely and effectively emits, reflects and refracts far infrared rays deep into the affected area of your hands. This treatment increases circulation at the molecular level, helping to deliver fresh nutrients and oxygenated blood to the arterioles (smallest blood arteries). Swelling is reduced, dormant cells are reactivated allowing the healing process to begin."

Case Studies

Case Studies: Summaries

Chillag, Shawn A. and Stephen Greenberg. "An Unusual Cause of Trigger Finger." *The New England Journal of Medicine,* 2011 (365) 7.

This case presented in a 62-year-old left-handed man. His fourth finger snapped painfully and locked up frequently, especially while writing. In technical terms, he suffered from a subluxation of the extensor digitorum tendon, commonly known as boxer's knuckle. The patient had not, however, experienced any trauma to his hand.

Boxer's knuckle results from an injury that weakens the tendon that straightens the finger joint -- the extensor tendon. Generally the injury is a tear. It typically occurs on the long finger, and the normal cause is a blow or repeated blows to the knuckle. It is a common injury for boxers and practitioners of the martial arts.

Rheumatoid arthritis can also cause disruption of the action of the extensor tendon, but inflammatory joint disease was ruled out in this case. Surgery was suggested, but the patient declined. After one year, there was no improvement.

———

Dala-Ali, Benan M., Amir Nakhdjevani, Mary A. Lloyd, Frederik B. Schreuder. "The Efficacy of Steroid Injection in the Treatment of Trigger Finger." *Clinics in Orthopedic Surgery,* 2012 (4) 263-268.

This study was conducted over a one-year period, with ninety individual trigger fingers receiving treatment via steroid injection. The results indicated that 66% of the digits were effectively treated. There was no statistical relationship between efficacy of the injection and the severity of the case or the presence or absence of a nodule at the base of the affected finger.

———

Degreef, I., R. Sciot and L. De Smet, "Delayed Post-Traumatic Trigger Finger in a 14-Year-Old Boy After Blunt Trauma: A Case Report." *Acta Chirurgica Belgica (ACB),* 2007 (107) 731-732.

In this case, a 14-year-old boy presented with a prominent palmar nodule affecting the middle finger of his left hand with progressive flexion. Six months earlier, he had fallen onto his outstretched hand, suffering a greenstick fracture of the distal radius, which was put in a cast for a month.

Surgical exploration revealed a nodule restricting the A1 pulley. The nodule was lying on and in the superficial flexor tendon. After surgery, the boy regained full motion in two weeks, and six months later there was no recurrence of the triggering.

Trigger finger resulting from blunt trauma of this kind is unusual. Reported cases typically involve a laceration or puncture wound. In this case, the force of the fall led to a chronic inflammation and the formation of the calcifying nodule, which progressed over time to a full-blown case of trigger finger.

———————

Divecha, H.M., J.V. Clarke, A. Coyle, S.J. Barnes. "Experience From a 'One-Stop' Trigger Finger Clinic: A Report of Outcomes Following Corticosteroid Injection." *The Internet Journal of Hand Surgery*, 2012 (3) 2. DOI:10.5580/2bf2

This study set out with two goals, to determine if doctors (specifically general practitioners) accurately diagnose trigger finger, and how successfully the condition can be addressed with a course of two steroid injections.

Between September 2005 and November 2008, 200 cases of trigger finger were identified in a so-called "one-stop" trigger finger clinic located in a general hospital district. The study included a one-year follow up on each patient.

The researchers determined that GPs correctly referred trigger finger patients 94% of the time. Of those, 74% saw their issue resolved with one injection; 84% with two injections. Only 15% of patients required surgical intervention.

The patients who were 8.3 years younger than the average for the group were the most likely to see instances of recurrence.

The study concluded that in 84% of all cases, two steroid injections resolved trigger finger without recurrence. The injection method was judged a viable trigger finger treatment with the potential to greatly reduce the patient burden for upper limb specialists since the shots can be administered in a primary care setting.

Goshtasby, Parviz Hiroshi, Dale R. Wheeler, and Owen J. Moy. "Risk Factors for Trigger Finger Occurrence After Carpal Tunnel Release." *Hand Surgery*, 2010 (15) 2: 81-87.

This study examined 792 patients who underwent carpal tunnel release surgery. Because carpal tunnel and trigger finger are common ailments treated by hand surgeons, the researchers were attempting to determine the risk of new onset trigger finger following carpal tunnel surgery.

The results indicated new onset in 6.3% of cases, or 50 out of 792. The two variables that seemed to point to an increased risk were the presence of osteoarthritis, and the use of endoscopic procedures to relieve the carpal tunnel.

Researchers concluded that based on these results, the potential for new onset trigger finger should be discussed with patients before endoscopic carpal tunnel release is performed.

It should be noted that there is no known correlation between carpal tunnel and trigger finger in the initial onset of either condition.

———————

Harb, Ziad, Quamar Bismil, and David M. Ricketts. "Trigger Finger Presenting Secondary to Leiomyoma: A Case Report." *Journal of Medical Case Reports* (2009) 3:7284.

In this case, a right-handed Caucasian male office worker, age 39, presented with a three-month history of trigger finger on his right ring finger with locking and clicking. A tender mass was also present, but the lump was larger than typical with a Notta's nodule.

When ultrasound was used, an elliptical soft tissue mass was detected and subsequently removed during surgery. It proved to be a spindle-celled stromal lesion consistent with leiomyoma.

A leiomyoma is a benign mass of smooth muscle material that rarely becomes a malignant tumor. The authors of the study could find no reference in the relevant literature to the presence of a leiomyoma causing a trigger digit.

In their conclusion, the authors wrote, "As we demonstrate with this case, uncommon pathology may present in a relatively common condition. We advise careful and methodical assessment of patients presenting with trigger finger, because although the majority of cases will be routine and uncomplicated, there are rare occasions when an underlying tumor is the cause of symptoms."

Lee, Young-Keun, Byung-Sup Kam, Kwang-Won Lee, Whoan-Jeang Kim, and Won-Sik Choy. "Ten Trigger Fingers in an Adult Man: A Case Report." *Journal of Korean Medical Science*, 2007 (22) 170-172.

The subject of this study was a 39-year-old man who developed trigger finger in all ten digits over a three-month period. He had a lifelong history of tingling in his hands during cold weather, with a bluish discoloration of his fingers.

When the man began working six days of the week with vibrating tools requiring a forceful grip, the problems in his hands intensified. Both his mother and a maternal aunt had been treated surgically for multiple trigger fingers.

Obvious nodules were present on both hands affecting the thumb, middle, and ring fingers. Surgery was performed on all ten fingers. The researchers believed the man suffered from Raynaud's Syndrome, which is a vasopastic disorder causing discoloration of the fingers and toes, but they were unable to arrive at a definitive determination.

The doctors did, however, conclude that the nature of the man's work, the genetic history of trigger finger, and the likely presence of Raynaud's Syndrome explained the locking of all ten fingers simultaneously.

Marcus, Alexander M., James E. Culver, Jr., and Thomas R. Hunt III. "Treating Trigger Finger in Diabetics Using Excision of the Ulnar Snap of the Flexor Digitorum Superficialis with or without A1 Pulley Release." *American Association of Hand Surgery*, 2007 (2) 227-231.

This study looked at both the short and long-term effectiveness of trigger finger release in diabetic patients. It is often difficult to restore motion and to eliminate trigger in diabetic patients because in severe cases, diabetics tend to have thick, stiff hands.

Their conclusion was that for diabetics, excision of the ulnar slip of the flexor digitorum superficialis with or without A1 pulley release was both safe and effective. Surgeons who perform A1 release without the ulnar slip should feel comfortable adding the additional work when they believe the tendon may not glide through a full arc of motion with the typical pulley release only.

Nakagawa, Akiko, Tetsuji Yamamoto, Toshihiro Akisue, Takashi Marui, Toshiaki Hitora, Teruya Kawamoto, Tetsuya Nakatani, Keiko Nagira, Shinichi Yoshiya, and Masahiro Kurosaka. "Trigger Finger Due to a Tendon Sheath Fibroma." *SICOT Online Report* E025. 2003.

In this case, an 86-year-old woman presented with triggering of her right middle finger that had been going on for a month. For the year prior, she had experienced a painless swelling over the metacarpophalangeal joint of the finger.

Following magnetic resonance imaging (MRI), a lesion was visible on the flexor tendon sheath. Surgical excision was performed, and the mass proved to be a benign soft tissue fibroma. The researchers discovered only eight other cases in the literature where a trigger finger was caused by a soft tissue tumor.

———————

Pampliega, T. and A.J. Arenas. "An Unusual Trigger Finger." *Acta Orthopaedic Belgica*, 1997 (63) 2.

In this case, a 16-year-old girl could not extend the middle finger of her left hand. When she attempted to do so, she heard and felt a "snapping" sensation accompanied by pain in her wrist. During surgery, doctors found the tendon sheath to be enlarged, and a benign fatty lipoma tumor was present in the wrist. Eighteen months later, a second surgery was performed when the girl complained of pain near the scar that occurred when she bent her fingers and wrist. The doctors were concerned that the tumor had grown back. Instead, they found a mass of scar tissue roughly the size of a pea. The adhesion was removed, and precautions were taken during physiotherapy to prevent its recurrence. Trigger fingers caused by tumors are rare, as are second surgeries to address the problem. In this case, triggering originated from a benign tumor in the wrist, making the case all the more unusual.

———————

Rottgers, Stephen A., Davis Lewis, and Ronit A. Wollstein. "Concomitant Presentation of Carpal Tunnel Syndrome and Trigger Finger." *Journal of Brachial Plexus and Peripheral Nerve Injury*, 2009 (4) 13.

This study looked at 108 participants with carpal tunnel syndrome and/or trigger finger as characterized by tenderness at the A1 pulley, clicking, catching, and locking. Carpal tunnel syndrome was identified by tingling and numbness in a median nerve distribution, motor and sensory nerve loss, a positive result on either a Phalen's or Tinsel's test, and positive electrophysiologic studies.

The average age of the participants was 62.2 years. Of those, 62% had carpal tunnel syndrome, and 38% had some degree of trigger finger. When evaluated as a total group, 61% showed signs of both conditions concurrently. Of that group, 53% suffered from diabetes.

While the study did conclude that it is common for carpal tunnel syndrome and trigger finger to occur at the same time, one of the conditions will be more pronounced than the other. The researchers posited a common local mechanism responsible for both conditions, but they did not find a conclusive link to diabetes.

––––––––––

Sternfield, M., E. Lipskier, Y. Finkelstein, A. Eliraz, and I. Hod. "Trigger Finger Relieved by Activation of Distal Ahshi Points in the Area of the Pericardium and Heart Meridians: A Pilot Study." *American Journal of Acupuncture*, 1991 (19) 319-322.

In this study, nine patients with trigger finger exhibiting impeded movement were referred for surgery when other therapies failed. They were treated with acupuncture points on the affected finger to a depth of 1-3 mm. The needles were left in for 30 minutes two times a week.

Seven of the nine in the study were reported as having been "cured." They experienced only moderate pain during the day, and had no functional disturbance. All underwent from 4 to 8 treatments. The follow-up period for the study was 4 to 12 months.

Additional References

American Academy of Orthopaedic Surgeons. "Trigger Finger." Orthoinfo.aaos.org. http://orthoinfo.aaos.org/topic.cfm?topic=a00024 (Accessed February 2013).

Bodor, Marko and Tiffany Flossman. "Ultrasound-Guided First Annular Pulley Injection for Trigger Finger." Journal of Ultrasound in Medicine, 2009 (28) 737-743.

Bond, Annie B. "13 Symptoms of Chronic Dehydration." Care2.com. http://www.care2.com/greenliving/13-symptoms-of-chronic-dehydration.html (Accessed February 2013).

Bowers, Elizabeth Shimer. "Gout and Diabetes." WebMD.com. http://arthritis.webmd.com/features/gout-and-diabetes (Accessed March 2013).

Chammas, Michel, Phillippe Bousquet, Eric Renard, Jean-Luc Poirier, Claude Jaffiol, Yves Allieu. "Dupuytren's Disease, Carpal Tunnel Syndrome, Trigger Finger, and Diabetes Mellius." *The Journal of Hand Surgery*, 1995 (20) 1: 109-114.

Cleveland Clinic. "Trigger Finger and Trigger Thumb Fundamentals." my.clevelandclinic.org. http://my.clevelandclinic.org/disorders/trigger_finger/or_over view.aspx, (Accessed December 2012).

CNN Health. "Trigger Finger." CNN.com. http://www.cnn.com/HEALTH/library/trigger-finger/DS00155.html (Accessed November 2012).

David Lincoln Nelson, M.D. Board Certified Hand Surgeon. "Cortisone Injection." davidhelson.md . http://www.davidlnelson.md/articles/Cortison_Injections.htm (Accessed March 2013).

The Electronic Textbook of Hand Surgery. "Clinical Example: Congential Trigger Thumb." EatonHand.com. http://www.eatonhand.com/img/img00069.htm (Accessed March 2013).

Flatt, Adrian F. "Notta's Nodules and Trigger Digits." *Proceedings* (Baylor University of Medicine), 2007 April. (20:2) 143-145.

Fleisch, S.B., K.P. Spindler, and D.H. Lee. "Corticosteroid Injections in the Treatment of Trigger Finger: A Level I and II Systematic Reivew." Journal of the American Academy of Orthopaedic Surgeons, 2007 (15) 166-171.

Gellman, Harris. Acupuncture Treatment for Musculoskeletal Pain: A Textbook for Orthopedics, Anesthesia, and Rehabilitation. CRC Press: 2002.

Guerini, Henri, Eric Pessis, Nicolas Theumann, Janine-Sophie Le Quintrec, Raphael Campagna, Alain Chevrot, Antoine Feydy, and Jean-Luc Drape. "Sonographic Appearance of Trigger Fingers." *Journal of Ultrasound Medicine*, 2008 (27) 1407-1413.

Huntley, A. "The Skin and Diabetes Mellitus." Dermatology Online Journal. Dermatology.cdlib.org. http://dermatology.cdlib.org/DOJvol1num2/diabetes/hand.html (Accessed February 2013).

Hyman, Mark. "How Diet Soda Makes You Fat (And Other Food and Diet Industry Secrets). HuffingtonPost.com.

http://www.huffingtonpost.com/dr-mark-hyman/diet-soda-health_b_2698494.html (Accessed March 2013).

Lab Tests Online. "Synovial Fluid Analysis." LabTestOnline.org. http://labtestsonline.org/understanding/analytes/synovial/tab/test (Accessed January 2013).

Mayo Clinic. "Trigger Finger." MayoClinic.com. http://www.mayoclinic.com/health/trigger-finger/DS00155 (Accessed December 2012).

McVitamins: A Health Information Site. "Our Need for Water." McVitamins.com. http://www.mcvitamins.com/water.htm (Accessed March 2013).

Medscape. "Physical Medicine and Rehabilitation for Trigger Finger." emedicine.medscape.com. http://emedicine.medscape.com/article/328996-overview (Accessed March 2013).

Mount Sinai Hospital. "Trigger Finger." MountSinai.com. "Trigger Finger." http://www.mountsinai.org/patient-care/health-library/diseases-and-conditions/trigger-finger (Accessed March 2013).

NHS Choices. "Trigger Finger." NHS.uk. http://www.nhs.uk/conditions/Trigger-finger/Pages/Introduction.aspx (Accessed January 2013).

Peters-Veluthamaningal, C., J.C. Winters, K.H. Groenier, and B. Meyboom-de Jong. "Corticosteroid Injections Effective for Trigger Finger in Adults in General Practice: A Double Blind Randomized Placebo Controlled Trial." Annals of the Rheumatic Diseases, 2008 (67) 1262-1266.

Quinnell, RC. "Conservative Management of Trigger Finger." *Practitioner*, 1980 (224) 187-90.

Saldana, Miguel J. "Trigger Digits: Diagnosis and Treatment." *Journal of the American Academy of Orthopaedic Surgeons*, 2001 (9) 246-252.

Singh, Vivek Ajit, S.T.B. Chong, S. Marriapan. "Trigger Finger: Comparative Study Between Corticosteroid Injection and Percutaneous Release." *The Internet Journal of Orthopedic Surgery*, 2006 (3) 2. DOI: 10.5580/889.

Scopelliti, A.R. "Sugar, A Neurotoxin?" Jersey Shore Regional Center for Vertigo, Dizziness, Dystonia and ADD and ADHD. Dcneuro.net. http://www.dcneuro.net/vertigo/sugar-a-neurotoxin (Accessed March 2013).

Wang, Denise. "Nonsurgical Exercises & Rehab for Trigger Finger." Livestrong.com. http://www.livestrong.com/article/434590-nonsurgical-exercises-rehab-for-trigger-finger/ (Accessed March 2013).

WebMD. "What Does Rheumatoid Arthritis Do to My Body?" WebMD.com. http://www.webmd.com/rheumatoid-arthritis/what-does-rheumatoid-arthritis-do-to-my-body (Accessed February 2013).

WebMD. "Arthritis and Trigger Finger." WebMD.com. http://www.webmd.com/osteoarthritis/guide/trigger-finger (Accessed February 2013).

Wei, Nathan, M.D. "Trigger Finger and Massage." Arthritis-Treatment-and-Relief.com. http://www.arthritis-treatment-and-relief.com/trigger-finger-massage.html (Accessed December 2012).

Glossary

A

Active Release Technique (ART) - A system of soft tissue, movement-based massage used by chiropractors to treat issues with the muscles, tendons, ligaments, fascia, and nerves. It was developed and patented by P. Michael Leahy.

acupuncture - A system of complementary medicine that involves pricking the skin or tissues with needles. Most commonly used to relieve pain. Has its origins in Eastern medical philosophy, especially that originating in China.

amyloidosis - A rare disease resulting from the build-up of amyloid proteins in the organs, usually produced by the bone marrow. Amyloidosis frequently affects the heart, kidneys, liver, spleen, nervous system, and gastrointestinal tract.

asymptomatic - Exhibiting no symptoms of a previously present condition.

Azithromycin - An antibacterial medication sold under the trade name Zithromax.

B

bilateral - Having or relating to both sides of a thing. In medical terms, a condition that occurs simultaneously on both sides of the body.

C

carpal tunnel syndrome - A painful condition of the hand and fingers caused by the compression of a major nerve in the wrist where it passes over the carpal bones. This is one of the most frequently diagnosed repetitive stress injuries in the United States.

chiropractic - The diagnosis and manipulative treatment of misalignments of the joints, especially those present in the spinal column.

clostridium histolyticum - A bacterium found in wounds, where it induces necrosis of tissue by producing a cytolytic exotoxin.

congenital - A disease or a physical abnormality present from birth.

corticosteroid - A synthetic steroid used in treating inflammatory and allergic diseases.

cortisone - A synthetic form of a naturally occurring hormone used to treat rheumatoid arthritis, allergic and skin disease, and inflammation.

cumulative trauma disorder - A disorder in which a part of the body is repeatedly injured by overuse.

D

dehydration - In medical terms, a condition caused by the excessive loss of water from the body, which causes sodium levels to rise in the blood. Dehydration is most often caused by excessive sweating. Vomiting, and diarrhea, and electrolyte deficiency occurs rapidly. If left untreated, the body goes into shock, and death can result.

De Quervain's Disease - Originally known as washerwoman's sprain, this condition is caused by inflammation of the tendon attached to the thumb, causing pain that radiates upwards into the lower arm.

diabetes - A medical condition in which the pancreas fails to produce adequate levels of insulin. As a result, glucose in the blood cannot be absorbed by the body's cells. Symptoms include frequent urination, lethargy, thirst (in excess), and hunger.

diclofenac - A nonsteroidal anti-inflammatory drug taken to reduce inflammation and as an analgesic for pain. It is sold under a variety of trade names.

diffuse - In medical terms, diffuse means not definitively limited or localized.

Dupuytren's Contracture - A disease of the fibrous tissue of the palm lying between the skin and the underlying tendons. The tissues thicken progressively, and as they tighten, the palm contracts, drawing the fingers inward.

E

endoscope - An instrument for examining the interior of a bodily structure in a minimally invasive way.

epicondylitis - A painful, often disabling inflammation of the muscle and tissue of the elbow due to repetitive stress on the forearm. Commonly known as "tennis elbow."

epilepsy - A neurological disorder marked by sudden and recurrent episodes of sensory disturbance, loss of consciousness, or convulsions.

ergonomic - An adjective referring primarily to workplace design intended to provide optimum comfort while avoiding stress or injury.

erythrocyte sedimentation rate - The rate at which red blood cells settle out in a tube of blood under standardized conditions. A high rate normally indicates the presence of inflammation.

Ethambutol - A bacteriostatic antimycobacterial drug usually prescribed to treat tuberculosis.

extensor muscles - Muscles whose contractions extend or stretch a body part.

F

fascia - In anatomical terms, a sheet or band of fibrous connective tissue enveloping, separating, or binding together muscles, organs, and other soft structures of the body.

fibroma - A benign fibrous tumor of connective tissue.

fixed deformity - A permanent or semi-permanent state of bodily malformation, distortion, or disfigurement.

flexor muscles - Muscles whose contractions bend a joint.

G

glucose - A simple sugar that is an important energy source in living organisms. The main type of sugar in the blood, and the major source of energy for the body's cells.

gout - A disease in which defective metabolism of uric acid causes acute pain in joints, especially those of the feet.

Graston Technique - A therapeutic method for diagnosing and treating disorders of the skeletal muscles and related connective tissues employing six stainless steel tools to detect and resolve adhesions.

I

ibuprofen - A nonsteroidal anti-inflammatory drug used in the treatment of fever, headaches, arthritic pain, muscle aches, and menstrual cramps.

L

lactate dehydrogenase - An enzyme that catalyzes the conversion of lactate to pyruvate, which is an important step in the production of energy in cells.

ligament - A short band of tough, flexible, fibrous connective tissue that connects two bones or cartilages, or holds together a joint.

lipoma – A benign tumor of fatty tissue

M

Mycobacterium kansaii - A bacterium that causes a pulmonary disease that resembles tuberculosis.

N

naproxen - A nonsteroidal anti-inflammatory drug used primarily in the management of arthritis and as a painkiller.

neuralgia - Intense, typically intermittent pain that travels along the path of a nerve, especially in the head or face.

neuroma - Any tumor that develops from cells in the body's nervous system.

nodule - A small swelling or aggregation of cells in the body, especially an abnormal one.

non-Newtonian fluid - A fluid whose flow properties are not described by a single constant value of viscosity.

Notta's Nodule - A palpable nodule affecting the A1 pulley of a digit affected with "trigger finger." These nodules were discovered by A. Notta in 1850.

NSAID - The generally accepted acronym for "nonsteroidal anti-inflammatory drug."

O

osteoarthritis - A degenerative joint disease, which destroys the joint cartilage and underlying bone.

P

percutaneous - Made, done, or effected through the skin.

R

Raynaud's Syndrome - A vasopastic disorder causing discoloration of the fingers, toes, and occasionally other areas of the body. The nails may become brittle, with longitudinal ridges, and the fingers often turn blue.

repetitive stress injury - Injuries of the musculoskeletal and nervous system caused by repetitive tasks, forceful exertions, vibrations, mechanical compressions (pressing against hard surfaces), or sustained awkward positions.

rheumatoid arthritis - A systemic inflammatory disease manifesting in multiple joints, primarily affecting the synovium membrane leading to the erosion of both cartilage and bone, with resulting pain, swelling, and deformity.

Rifampin - An antibiotic used primarily in the treatment of tuberculosis and leprosy.

S

sonography - Diagnostic medical sonography, or ultrasound, uses high frequency sound to create images of specific areas of the body for diagnostic purposes.

stenosing tenosynovitis - A progressive restriction of the sheath surrounding a tendon at the base of a finger or thumb with resulting inflammation and interruption of motion. Commonly called "trigger finger."

synovium - A thin membrane in snovial or freely moving joints that lines the capsule of the joint and secretes lubricating synovial fluid.

synovial fluid - The lubricating fluid secreted by the membrane lining joints and tendon sheaths.

systemic - Pertaining to or affecting the body as a whole.

T

tendon - A flexible, but inelastic cord of strong fibrous collagen tissue attaching a muscle to a bone.

tendon sheath - A layer of membrane around a tendon, which permits the tendon to move.

tendonitis - The inflammation of a tendon.

U

uric acid - The water-insoluble end product of primate purine metabolism. The deposit of uric acid as crystals in the joints and kidneys causes gout.

V

viscosity - The state of being thick, sticky, and semi-fluid in consistency. The property of a fluid that resists the force tending to cause the fluid to flow. In rough terms, the "consistency" of a fluid expressed commonly as "thick" or "thin."

About Author

Joshua L Sho is an online entrepreneur, author and researcher, with science background. As a hobby, he plays the piano skillfully and he has keen interest in teaching the intermediate to advanced level piano players. As an online business person, Joshua spends most of his working hours on the computer and mobile devices which was one of the reasons he suffered with trigger finger.

Joshua wrote this book out of his passion to help others, and also because he loves to research and share knowledge on many topics of interest to him and his online community.

Joshua has made every effort to be as thorough, unbiased and objective as possible in presenting the facts and interpreting his findings on this topic.

For further queries regarding any aspect of this book, you can reach him on his email;

Joshua@TriggerFingerCure.com

Dedication

This comprehensive guide and toolkit is dedicated to all trigger finger and pain in the thumb sufferers. This is to your health and happiness.

Index

flexor tendon 35, 41

tendon sheath 28, 29, 37

tendonitis 13

tennis elbow 13

thyroid 16, 35

(see also hypothyroidism)

trigger finger

associated conditions 34-35

case studies 16-17, 31-32, 33-34, 38, 42, 44-45, 69-77

causes 27-31

chiropractic treatment 43-45

classic 11, 12, 14, 18, 19, 20, 29, 32, 36, 47, 54

diagnosis 24-25, 48-50

diffuse 12, 53

exercises 40-41

grades 24

products 66-68

references 65-66

risk factors 32-33

mechanics 19

stages 24

symptoms 20-24

thumb 35 (congenital)

treatment 36-46

tuberculosis 35, 55

CPSIA information can be obtained at www.ICGtesting.com
Printed in the USA
LVOW01s1658041013

355490LV00024B/1390/P

FEB 1 3 2016